MUDRAS

40 Powerful Hand Gestures To Unleash The Physical, Mental And Spiritual Healing Power In YOU!

Diane Clarke

© 2015

Contents

Introduction

Welcome! I'm truly delighted to share with you my exciting new book, "40 Powerful Hand Gestures To Unleash The Physical, Mental And Spiritual Healing Power In YOU!"

Despite the stress that surrounds our daily lives, we've all been through situations where we were "*pushed*" to experience moments of deep peace.

I say *pushed*, for we didn't go after these moments with intent. Heck, we didn't even know they existed within us! They happened at a time when we least expected; when we'd surrendered to the destiny that awaited us.

Consider this in your own life – perhaps a time when you were stuck in traffic with no hope of reaching home soon, or when you were bedridden and down with a nasty flu, having nothing to do or no one to talk to? These are your waiting periods.

They can be painfully aggravating, testing your very patience and will to continue. OR, they can be times of rejuvenation, when you are forced to go past your demons and re-discover yourself. These periods can bring about an inner shift that positively changes the way you see life. Suddenly, the packed traffic seems to ease up and clear a way for you. Your bed or the flu you've been stuck with for days doesn't trouble you anymore.

You find that the answer to all your problems resides INSIDE, and not outside of you!

You see, we possess the power to nurture our lives and destroy it too. Unfortunately, we've become so used to victimizing ourselves that we don't think we are ever capable of harming ourselves. It's a convenient idea we've trained our minds to believe in: *to reach out for external solutions and look for answers outside our body!*

This book urges you to seek answers from within, to endorse alternate therapies for healing and a better quality lifestyle. The practice of "Mudras" is one such holistic science and offers tremendous benefit at all levels of our being. In this book, I introduce this practice to you.

Here, you will learn about:
-*Yoga Mudras: simple hand gestures to effortlessly revitalize your body and mind!*

-Breathing and meditation techniques to accompany Mudra practice. Together, they can transcend you to a state of deep inner peace and fabulous well-being!
-Direct tips to elevate your OVERALL experience of life!

By practicing Mudras in combination with breathing and visualization techniques, I've been able to successfully heal myself from physical, mental and emotional struggles. I've also been able to powerfully overcome inner conflicts, and experience longer periods of peace and contentment. *I want you to experience this too!*

In fact, I've written this book with YOU in mind.

Through this book, you will discover that Mudras are universally:
-FREE! *Yes, you don't have to pay a dime for it!*
-Super convenient and can be practiced anytime, anyplace!
-Customized for YOU, so you get to decide what Mudra you want to practice, and when!
-A sure way to beat expensive treatments, over the counter medications and nasty medicinal side effects that we've gotten used to!
-A 5000-year old time-tested science, that WORKS!!

Intrigued?

I warmly welcome you to share my experience. As always, I've made this a "practical" guide. I urge you to try out the Mudras even as you read this book; you will be surprised and super enthusiastic at the results! ☺

~ Diane Clarke

Chapter 1 – The Science of Mudras

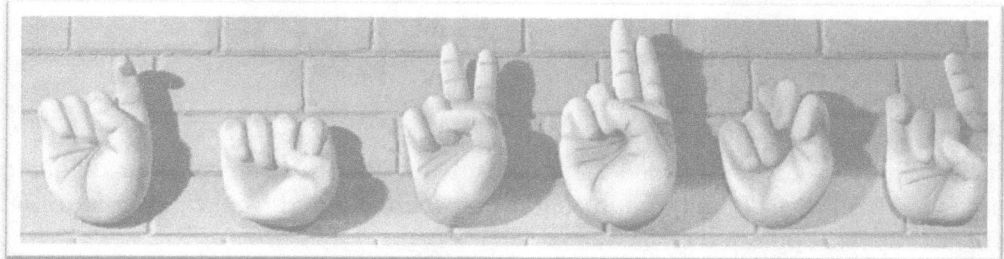

By Charles Haynes @ https://www.flickr.com/photos/haynes/2172995172/

In order to fully understand the effectiveness of practicing Mudras, we must first understand the connection between us, our hands, and the *5 elements* that reside within us. This chapter explains this connection, and explores the significance this has on our mind, body and spirit.

While some of you may find this a tad esoteric, pagan even, let me quickly assure you that this is not the case. The practice of Mudras is a clear *science*. I do encourage you to actively contemplate on this chapter as here lies the fundamental key to understanding this holistic practice.

Energy Consciousness and the Elements of Life

Consider these elemental questions about the Universe.

-Is there a conscious field of radiant energy that we are ALL made of?
-Are we interconnected to each other by this force of omnipresent energy?
-Does it exist outside of our body and does its effect have any impact on the way we function and live as human beings?

The answer is a resounding **"YES"**!!

Our ancestors seemed to have had it all figured out. A peek into ancient wisdom clearly echoes the nature of 5 essential elements, which exist *inside* and *amidst* us.
-Fire.
-Air.
-Space or Ether.
-Earth.
-Water.
When we make a conscious effort to understand the true *source* and nature of our existence, we can potentially recognize that the entire universe is made up of a collective force, consisting of these 5 elements.

Everything that resides within this universal space is a reflection of this force, us included!

Macrocosm in Microcosm

Ancient Indian seers understood the greatest truth of our existence: *"that all living things are an integral part of nature, that we were created from it, exist in it and will have to one day return to it!"*

What exists in, resides out!

According to the fundamental principles of these ancient beliefs, there is a definite connection and synchronicity between all that exists in the entire Cosmos and Universe, the *"Macrocosm"*, and us, the *"Microcosm"*.

We are made up of the same 5 elements that make up this magnificent Universe. These 5 elements are subtle states of matter and energy, interconnected to form the very core of our existence and everything that surrounds us. Hence, these elements also epitomize the multi-dimensional co-existence of Macrocosm and Microcosm!

Their presence and conscious state in the *Macrocosm* has a direct relationship on how they function inside us, in the *Microcosm*. Conversely, the essence of these elements within us, impacts the life outside us.

We ARE the 5 Elements!

Considering that our body is predominantly controlled by the cohabitation of these elements, in a sense, WE intrinsically BECOME the 5 ELEMENTS that exist within us! Our body therefore exhibits and expresses unique qualities that are symbolic to the dominating element present in it.

Understanding these traits can help us identify and subsequently heal any imbalance that resides within our body.

There's more.

Our fingers help *regulate* these 5 essential elements of life.

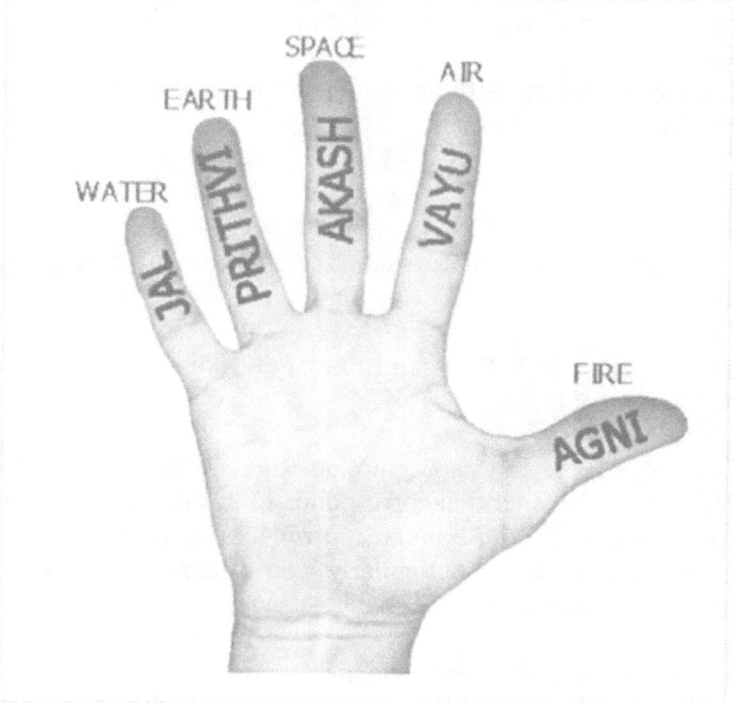

- The thumb controls the FIRE element in us.
- The index finger controls the AIR element in us.
- The middle finger controls the SPACE element in us.
- The ring finger controls the EARTH element in us.
- The little finger controls the WATER element in us.

Here then, lies the healing power of Mudras!

The key to human well-being lies in the harmonious coexistence of these five elements, *within* us.

In following sections of this chapter, we explore in thorough detail how each element affects and responds to the Universe, and us. This will form the basis for the rest of your learning, and help you effortlessly adapt an effective Mudra practice!

We are the EARTH!

Earth symbolizes the solid form of matter and epitomizes qualities of *longevity, strength* and *consistence* in us. Parts of our body that exhibit firmness and strength represent the earth element that resides within us. Nails, bones, teeth, hair, skin along with the sense of smell represent this form.

Our power to endure struggles with absolute resolve and conviction comes from the dominating earth element in our body.

We are WATER
The famous Zen master Suzuki once said, "*If you want to know your mind, just observe water*".

Water exemplifies that which flows and does not take shape. Its nature is free-flowing and cannot be controlled.

In the mind, it manifests feelings and emotions that are purely *impulsive* and *free-willed*. Just as water reflects all that corresponds to it, the mind too reflects all that traverses through its path. You cannot control a thought until you consciously meditate on drifting away from it. Similarly, you cannot force a change until the mind wants to embrace and permit the change!

Water is also a miraculous "life giver": it nourishes, hydrates and instills life into our body. It flows through our body while distributing nutrition, regulating its temperature and carrying away wastes. Body liquids such as blood, Lymph, urine and intracellular fluid are some of the physical forms of water present in our body.

When there is an imbalance in any of the above body liquids, it's likely that there is an imbalance in the water levels traversing through our bodies!

We are all that ignites light; we are the FIRE!
Fire has the power to *transform*, scorch and illuminate everything that it comes in contact with!

All that we consume through food and nutrition ultimately gets transformed into tissues and energies by the fire element present in our body. In the body, fire controls parts such as the heart, small intestine, adrenal glands, pancreas, liver, stomach, nervous system and bladder. An overdose of this element can result in inflammation of the joints, chronic infections and lung dryness. Excess heat can also cause sleep disorders, anxiety, restlessness and painful migraines.

Fire and its effects on the mind:
This element also controls factors in the brain that influence *perception*, and hence impacts the relationships we have with people. Fire is responsible for the love you feel for something or someone. Conversely, it can also be responsible for that

nervous feeling you have at the pit of your stomach, when you're anxious and know something is not right.

On a deeper level, Fire is that element that expresses itself as all things vibrant, loving and fulfilling. You see, we are inherently wired to feel the happiest when the fire element is in balance. The presence of warmth and sunshine almost instantly translates into feelings of love and togetherness with nature. Just as most birds thrive and venture out in summer and flowers blooms under sunlight, we too are designed to draw on the expansive warmth of fire for greater fulfillment!

We are the AIR that surrounds us!
As we speak, I ask you to draw attention to the air element within your body.

You'll notice the breath you just took in filled up your lungs, passed through your respiratory system, cleansed and *gave life to every cell in your body*! You'll also notice it carrying out unnecessary toxins and negative energy from your body to expel it into the space beyond!

Now, observe this element outside of you.

Do you feel its presence in the space that's around you? Do you see its propelling effect on trees, hear its reverberating buzz in your ear and feel it caress your skin?

Air is ALL that moves! It is dynamic and does not rest. Although you cannot see it, you feel its presence flow through every cell in your body, in every breath and step you take.

Air is that element that propels all that moves within us. Every movement in our body, be it the air we breathe, or the hands and legs we move is propelled by the air element in nature. Air controls the power of the mind and is responsible for the intellect, inspiration and imagination we exhibit. It is that masculine element which governs the four winds. It is that supreme energy that passes through all living and non-living things, filling life and movement into everything it touches!

Understanding the presence of air in your body can help you lead an energetic, vigorous, and healthier life!

We are ETHER!
Observe the rhythmic flow of air going in and leaving out of your body. Where does it come from and where does it go? If it comes from the space that exists amidst us and expels in to the space that is beyond, are we not a part of the space that provides and expels the very breath of our life?

YES! We are the empty SPACE!

Ether is the space in which everything happens. It is the space that distances the other four elements. It is the empty space that resides inside the body and that which prevails outside of it. Everything we know exists, resides in space and all that we don't, settles into it!

Understanding and regulating the levels of ether in your body will help you stay integrated with it.

When there is an imbalance in this element, the body degenerates and the elements flee their boundaries, giving rise to a number of health concerns.

Chapter 2 – Our Fingertips Are the Doorway to Balance

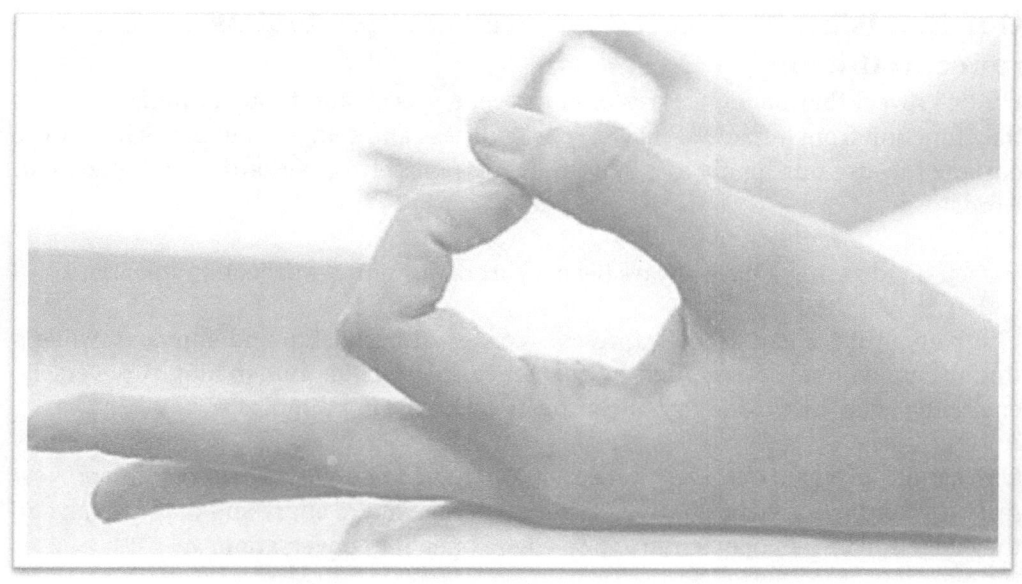

Source: http://i.ytimg.com/vi/IORed2wdc5g/maxresdefault.jpg

Our hands are a source of incredible power!

The human hand is more than the physical attributes we see and feel. Consisting of 27 bones and 15 joints all harmoniously working together, they are a source of tremendous power, capable of wielding intense dexterity and purpose!

This harmony plays a crucial role in our existence, and the experiences we seek as human beings. We can either use them as tools to facilitate the life WE want to lead, or use them to shape an outline of the world we want to be a part of.

On one side, they can nurture and heal LIFE. On the other, they can harm and destroy everything they've created! With such profound significance, *there's definitely more to our hands than meets the eye!*

Our hands stimulate and influence our thought patterns!

Our hands are an extension of our heart and are closely connected to our brain. This infers that every part of our hand has a reflexive connection to our brain, making it capable of engaging and influencing specific aspects in our brain.

Practicing symbolic hand movements or Mudras can help realign our thought process, revive our state of inner consciousness, and recognize its relationship with the entire cosmos!

Our hands are the sacred gateways to spiritual ascension and inner well-being!

Studies reveal that hand gestures often precede speech and thought, indicating that they function from a space of higher consciousness and self. It's almost as if we were designed to use our hands as a way to express ourselves, perhaps even better than words!

In fact, hand gestures have always been a part of our non-verbal communication!

Think about it - a handshake expresses feelings of friendship and approval, while a thumbs up symbol is regarded as the universal sign for hitchhiking. Conversely, encircling your thumb and forefinger together can mean a simple Ok.

Our hand movements can also reflect our state of mind and *reveal our inner most feelings*. For instance, a clenched fist indicates that you're angry and ready to take up the cudgels, while an open palm shows you're open for conversation.

They come naturally to us, and emphasize *deeper meaning* when we speak.

Here then lies the purpose of hand gestures, or Mudras.

What ARE Mudras?

Are they simply...

-Hand gestures or symbols that seal and stimulate the energy points between fingers?

OR

-Mystical positions that lead you to a state of higher consciousness and self-realization?

If only the answer was simple!

Mudras are all that is mentioned above and more - *To people who seek spiritual ascension; Mudras are revered as ancient sacred codes that connect with the mind, body and spirit!*

The power to heal resides within our hands!

When I recently mediated on the word "Mudra", I became consciously aware of its most popular physical form: the "chin Mudra", that which resembles the symbol of a lock.

This image stayed in my mind long enough to make me think of its significance. Metaphorically speaking, a lock conceals and masks a secret, a secret that is purposely kept hidden from all those who do not have the key to it: *to open the lock, you must first find its key!*

In comparison, our bodies are no different as they too consist of several locked passages. Through the course of stress and everyday drudgery, we end up blocking the flow of positive energy in our body, leading to a state of mental and physical disempowerment. Practicing regular Mudras can help heal and unblock any dysfunctional energy channels we might have created within our bodies!

We have the power to stay "Happy" and "dis-ease free"!

As discussed before, our body is made up of the five planetary *energies* that surround our cosmos. These five energies include:
- FIRE or *Agni*
- AIR or *Vayu*
- SPACE (Ether) or *Akasha*
- EARTH or *Prithvi*
- WATER or *Jal*

Human well-being lies in the harmonious coexistence of the five elements or energy points that resides within us. By *"tapping"* and *"unleashing"* chakras or special energy points in our body, we can stimulate trigger points to *unblock, heal* and *realign* ourselves. Through this experience, we enjoy greater health and well-being, draw deeper attention to our *inner self* and become one with our higher being!

In the end, understanding these closely guarded secrets while mastering the art of practicing Mudras can be the greatest gift you can give yourself.

Mudras work at every level of your being – mind, body and spirit. With regular practice, you can beat just about any disease or disorder! In fact, the next few chapters are loaded with therapeutic hand movements to heal disease – heart disease, digestive disorders, diabetes, poor immunity, low metabolism, obesity, poor stamina and low energy levels, mental restlessness, stress and anxiety – this list is potentially endless!

It's time we recognize the magnitude of this incredible power!

It's time we discover the significance of hand Mudras and the difference it can make to our lives. Remember that this is a process that can ultimately lead you to the hidden intelligence that guides the entire universe, us included.

It's time we practice and act on all that has been said! The time is NOW!

Chapter 3 – General Mudras for Everyday Living

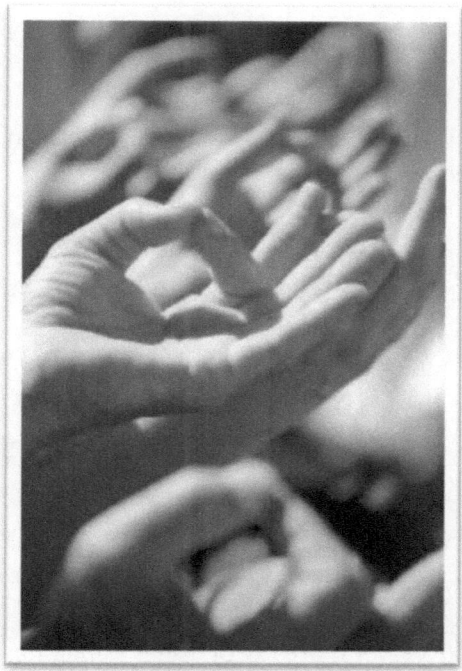

Source: http://www.3ho.org/kundalini-yoga/Mudra

Practicing Mudras everyday can successfully lead you to the path of supreme health and inner happiness. The ultimate goal is to cleanse your system, such that you live life in light and with clarity. With this section I introduce you to Mudras for everyday life and well-being.

Practice Guidelines

Before we jump into the Mudras, I'd like to share a few tips for a richer and more fulfilling experience:

- Mudras work best when practiced during or immediately after meditation. If time permits, practice Mudras after 15 minutes of meditation as you are likely to feel more centered and balanced at this time. Remember that this is no strict rule to follow. All I insist is that you practice them at a time and space that is most convenient to you!

- For greater effect, visualize the colors of the rainbow entering your body as you practice Mudras. The rainbow is a symbol of good fortune and inner harmony. Each color has a specific effect on the mind and body and visualizing these colors can help you achieve the desired result with greater effect. This is also the basis for Chakra – color therapy, as indicated by the image below.

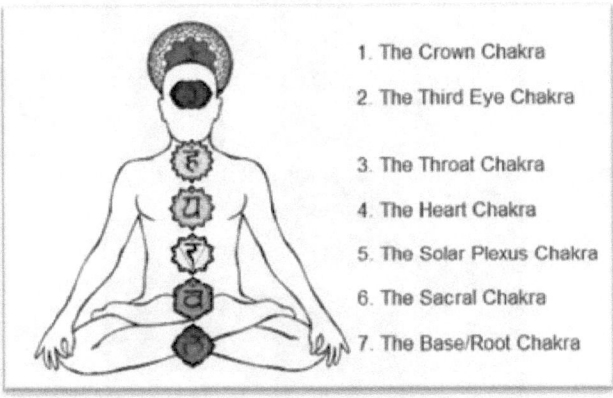

1. The Crown Chakra

2. The Third Eye Chakra

3. The Throat Chakra

4. The Heart Chakra

5. The Solar Plexus Chakra

6. The Sacral Chakra

7. The Base/Root Chakra

- Do not force control over your breath or inner thoughts. Instead, give into the experience and let them flow free. Your surrender will open up a whole new dimension to your experience, giving you something very special to hold onto at the end of the practice!

- Finally, remember that this is a learning process that will ultimately lead you to self-realization! *Make sure you own the Mudras while you practice them.*

- Feel free to come up with YOUR own guidelines as you grow and evolve through the practice.

Stay calm and enjoy the experience! ☺

Mudras for everyday life and well-being

JNANA MUDRA AND CHIN MUDRA

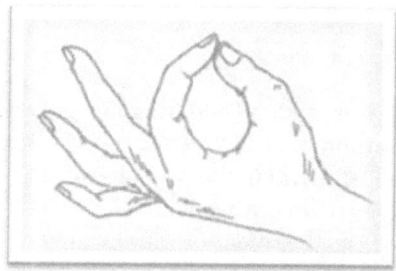

Instructions:
-Join the tip of your index finger with the tip of your thumb to form a circle.
-Stretch and straighten the remaining 3 fingers outwards.
-Place your hands on the knee with your fingers facing upwards.

Duration: This Mudra is known for its therapeutic benefits and can be practiced for as long as you can and want!

Benefits:
This Mudra focuses on realigning the flow of energy inwards, and to the mind in particular. It reduces mental conflicts such as inner chatter, restlessness and depression while promoting inner peace, superior concentration and mental agility.

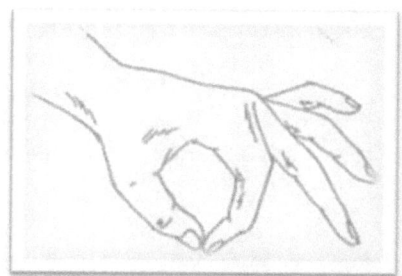

Note: A variation to this Mudra is the "Chin Mudra", in which you point your fingers downwards.

PRANA MUDRA

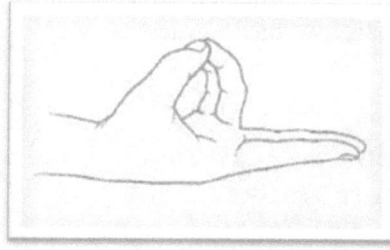

Instructions:
-Join the tips of your ring and little fingers with the tip of your thumb.
-Next, stretch and straighten the remaining 2 fingers such that they point outwards.
Duration: Practice this Mudra for as long as you can and want!

Benefits: Also known as the "Mudra of life", this Mudra nourishes energy, increases vitality, improves vision and works in co-ordination with other Mudras to aid good health and overall well-being.

Note: One of the key benefits of the Prana Mudra is its ability to make you feel rejuvenated and energized. This is also the reason it's used in combination with other Mudras: to increase their effectiveness on the mind and body.

APANA MUDRA

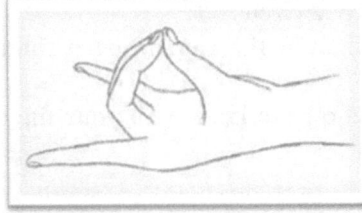

Instructions:
-Join the tips of your middle and ring fingers with the tip of your thumb.
-Next, stretch and straighten the remaining 2 fingers such that they point outwards.
Duration: This is a therapeutic Mudra and should be practiced for 45 minutes.

Benefits: Practicing this Mudra helps you connect with and utilize earth's energies to aid better digestion. It cleanses the entire body so as to remove toxins and strengthen it. In addition to this, it also regulates the process of excretion while reducing any burning sensation you might be suffering with.

ANJALI OR NAMASKARA MUDRA

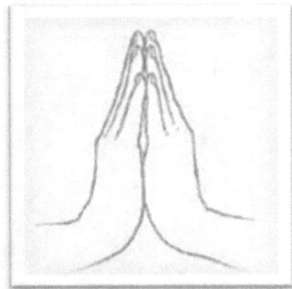

Instructions:
-Press your hands together with your palms facing each other and fingers pointed upwards.
-Bring it to the center of the chest and close to your heart chakra.
-Invoke feelings of gratitude and humility while recognizing the divine light force that exists in one another.
Duration: Practice this Mudra for as long as you can and want!

Benefits: Commonly seen as a way of greeting people in India, this Mudra touches a positive chord in the body, evoking feelings of oneness and togetherness with all those, around us. Practicing this Mudra regularly helps break through barriers of ego and selfishness while urging you to connect with the collective consciousness of every life-form that exists amongst us.

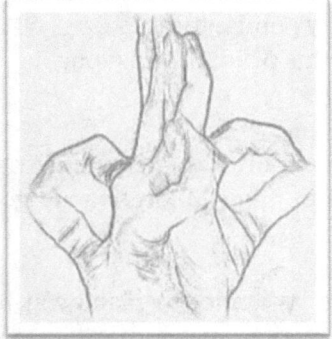

ABHAYA HRIDHIYA MUDRA OR COURAGEOUS HEART MUDRA

Instructions:
-Cross your right wrist over your left, with the back of the hands facing each other.

-Now, hook the right index finger around the left, middle right finger around the left, and the right little finger around the left.
-Next, stretch out and join your right ring finger with your right thumb. Repeat this step with your left ring finger and thumb.
-Finally, pull and draw in the root of the thumb to the base of your chest.
Duration: Practice this Mudra for as long as you can and want!

Benefits: This Mudra helps replace feelings of fear and apprehension with that of courage and self-belief. Practice this Mudra when you feel stressed and out of alignment. As this Mudra instantly connects with the heart chakra, it releases any knotted feelings of stress you might have inside.

PUSHPAPUTA MUDRA

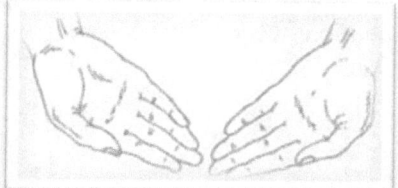

Instructions:
-Stretch your hands open such that they face each together.
-Let your palms stay open and facing upwards while you thumbs rest against the outer edge of your index fingers.
-Invoke feelings of openness and accept all that you are likely to experience.
Duration: Practice this Mudra for as long as you can and want!

Benefits: One only experiences what they attract from the universe. When you nurture feelings of gratitude and love, you attract similar experiences into your life. This Mudra symbolizes feelings of openness and acceptance. By practicing this Mudra regularly, you consciously bring about an inner shift in you: you therefore stay gratified for all the great things you have and express feelings of compassion and concern towards others. Ultimately, this inner shift transcends you to a state that attracts similar positive experiences.

VARUNA MUDRA

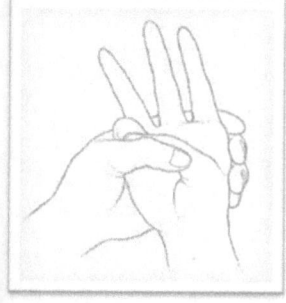

Instructions:
-Join the tip of your right little finger to the tip of your right thumb.
-Stretch and straighten out the remaining 3 fingers such that they face upwards.
-Wrap your left hand around the back of your right palm.
-Cradle you left thumb on the back of your right little finger and thumb.
Duration: This is a therapeutic Mudra and should be practiced for 45 minutes.

Benefits: Varuna Mudra controls and regulates the water metabolism in your body. Practicing this Mudra regularly can help reduce drying of eyes and skin. It also helps pacify Anemia, purifies blood, ease out painful cramps, regulate hormonal imbalance and cure skin allergies.

Note: As your body heals and responds to the therapeutic effects of this Mudra, you will notice your skin glow with tenderness and radiance!

PANKAJ MUDRA

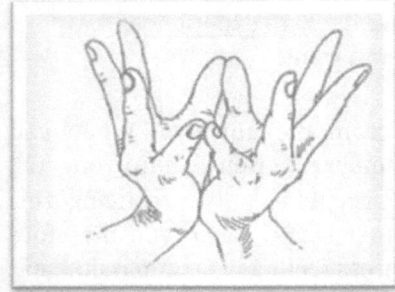

Instructions:
-Join your two palms such that they face each other.
-Next, join the two thumbs and little fingers
-Finally, stretch out the remaining 6 fingers (3 on each side) so as to resemble a blooming flower (lotus).
Duration: Practice this Mudra for as long as you can and want!

Benefits: This Mudra is a symbol of purity and openness. When you meditate in this Mudra, your mind becomes pure and uncluttered from the unnecessary baggage it carried before. On a physical level, this Mudra pacifies fever and regulates any irregularity in sleep patterns.

Chapter 4 – Mudras for Peak Physical Health

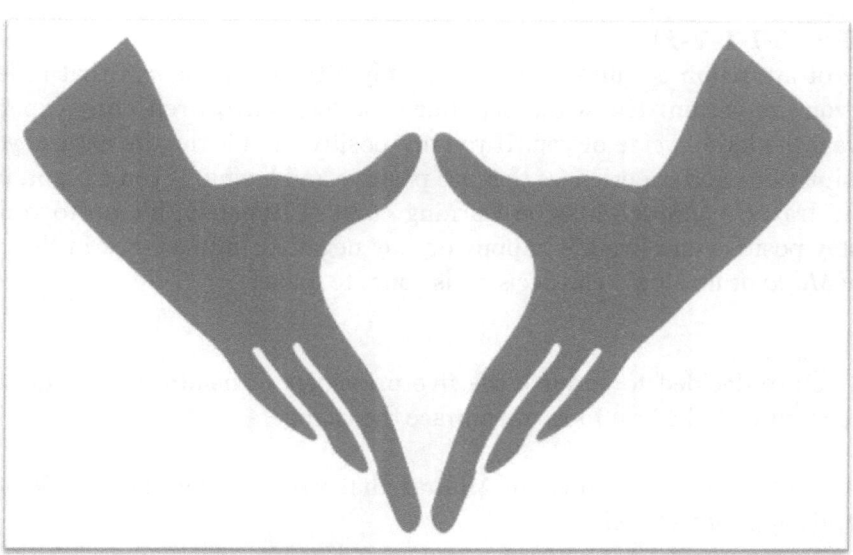

The Five Principles of Health
Following the five principles of health can see us leading a long, healthy and happy life. These principles work at regulating key factors that aid both, physical and mental well-being.

Eat Healthy!
Consuming a nutritious and balanced diet is one of the first steps to superior health and faster healing. Plate-up a generous share of fresh fruits and vegetables (preferably eaten raw). Make sure you also include foods such as cereals, milk, pulses as they work at giving you the balanced nutrition you need.

Avoid drugs, smoking and alcohol.
Steer clear of alcohol, drugs and smoking as they are known to attract diseases, like "bees to honey".

Practice Mudras regularly!
We've already emphasized the significance of practicing Mudras and yoga daily. They work at cleansing and regulating imbalances in the body, and hence keep you away from the medicinal grid for the long haul. Alternatively, you can also combine Mudras and yogic exercises with a few outdoor sport routines or workout exercises.

RELAX: Stay calm and stress-free!
Don't waste time in mulling over the past or thinking about the future. Instead, stay aware and live in the PRESENT! Most often than not, your decision to drop all

worries will lead you to a healthier and more fulfilling life. Practicing Mudras is a great way to de-stress. Later chapters talks about specific Mudras for greater mental balance and peace.

Think P-O-S-I-T-V-E!
The law of attraction is quite simple: You only attract experiences that reflect the person you are within. The world acts like a perfect mirror, reflecting experiences that reveal the hidden side of you. If you are positive and loving by nature, you will attract situations and experiences that are positive and loving. If you are not, you are bound to traverse through a steep learning curve. Ultimately, it's up to you: "you either stay positive and live life happily or stay negative and be stuck in the gloomy phase of *Maya* or illusion". The decision is yours to make!

Well, if you've decided to endorse the five principles of health, you might as well equip yourself with the best tools to embrace the change!

I've put together a list of powerful Mudras that work at delivering peak physical health and superior well-being.

Well then, let's get started, shall we?

Mudras to balance the "Air" element in the body
This section highlights the significance of the air element, "VAYU", present in our body.

In simple translation, Vayu means "wind". So just as the wind outside us directs the flow of everything that moves, the Vayu element inside the body, directs the flow of our "Prana", also known as our "life force energy".

There are five specific Vayus:
- *Prana Vayu*
- *Apana Vayu*
- *Samana Vayu*
- *Vyana Vayu and*
- *Udana Vayu*

Together these Vayus help in creating a level of balance as it ranges in and around the body. On a physical level; this element helps regulate your digestive tract. On a conceptual level, it helps enhance creativity, clarity and self-expression!

The exercises below illustrate two specific Mudras in particular:

- The *Vayu Mudra* works at regulating the upward movement of air and covers organs that reside between your throat and abdomen.
- The *Apana Vayu Mudra* works at regulating the downward movement of air and covers organs that reside from center of the stomach, (naval) down to the lower extremities.

VAYU MUDRA

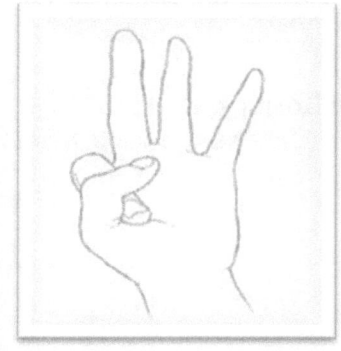

Instructions:
-Place the tip of your index finger at the base of your thumb.
-Next, gently cradle the thumb on the back of your index finger.
-Stretch and straighten out the remaining 3 fingers such that they point outwards.
Duration: Practice this Mudra for fifteen minutes to relieve any pain and discomfort caused due to flatulence and gastric problems. For chronic gastric conditions, practice this Mudra for 45 minutes. You can also split this up and practice it for 15 minutes, thrice a day.

Benefits: Vayu symbolizes the air element in the body. When there is an imbalance in the food we consume and the lifestyle we lead, there's every chance that there might be an increase in the air element within our body. Elevated levels of the air element can cause uncomfortable conditions such as flatulence, gastric pain and abdominal bloating. Practicing this Mudra can help regulate and eliminate any such conditions present in the body.

Note: While this Mudra effectively works at bringing down gastric concerns, it should **NOT BE** used as a substitute for medical treatment!

APANA VAYU MUDRA

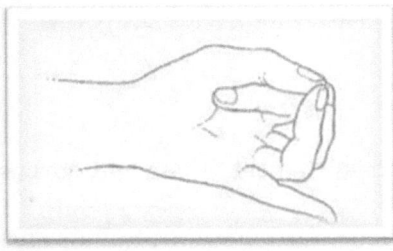

Instructions:
-In this Mudra, Place the tip of your index finger at the base of your thumb.
-Next, join the tip of the thumb with the tips of the middle and ring fingers.
-Stretch and straighten out your little finger such that it points outwards

Duration: Practice this Mudra for fifteen daily minutes to strengthen your heart. For chronic heart conditions, practice this Mudra for 45 minutes. You can also split this up and practice it for 15 minutes, thrice a day.

Benefits: This Mudra stimulates energy towards the heart chakra in the body. It's known for its miraculous effects in treating heart attacks, and is therefore known as "the lifesaver". When practiced regularly, this Mudra works at strengthening the heart and reduces risk from heart-related diseases.

Note: While this Mudra is known for its positive effect in treating heart attacks, it should NOT BE used as a substitute for medical treatment! Make sure you reach out for appropriate medical assistance in time.

Mudras for peak physical health
SURYA MUDRA

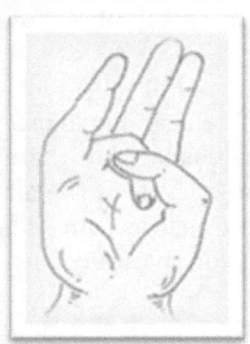

Instructions:
-Tuck the tip of your ring finger to the base of your thumb.
-Now, gently cradle your thumb on the back of your ring finger.
-Stretch and straighten out the remaining three fingers such that they point upwards.

Duration: Practice this for 45 minutes daily. You can also split this up by practicing it for 15 minutes, thrice a day.

Benefits: This Mudra works at regulating the "earth element" while increasing the "fire element" in the body. Practicing this Mudra regularly reduces progressive weight gain or obesity, regulates loss of appetite, constipation or indigestion, cures throat irritations such as cough and asthma, and pacifies high cholesterol in the body.

Note: As this Mudra increases the fire element in the body, it helps burn down fat deposits and is excellent for weight loss!

LINGA MUDRA

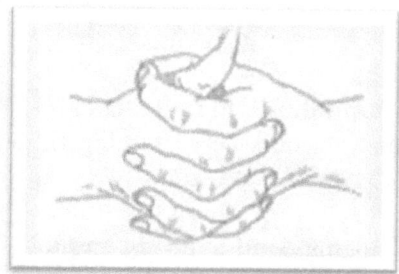

Instructions:
-First, bring your palms together, drawing them in front of you.
-Next, interlace your fingers, leaving your thumbs free and pointing upwards.
-Lastly, encircle your left thumb with the index and thumb of your right hand.

Duration: Practice this for 45 minutes daily. You can also split this up by practicing it for 15 minutes, thrice a day.

Benefits: The Linga Mudra works at increasing the fire element in the body. In this Mudra, we increase the heat element, and with it raise the levels of energy, present in the body. By practicing this Mudra regularly, you also gain access to the divine portal of cosmic energy. With it, you can re-direct some of the divine cosmic energy to flow into your body. Hence, it is also known as an energy-charging Mudra!

Note: This Mudra strengthens your immune system while making it resistant to common allergies and infections. Like the Surya Mudra, the Linga Mudra too increases the fire element in the body, making it an effective therapy for weight loss!

KIDNEY MUDRA

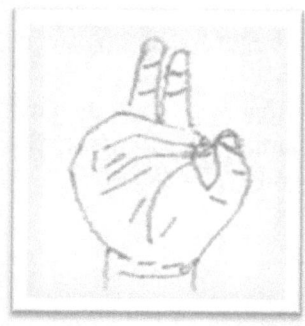

Instructions:
-Tuck in the tips of your little and ring fingers to the base of your thumb.
-Next, gently cradle the thumb on the back of your little and ring fingers.
-Stretch and straighten out the remaining 2 fingers such that they point outwards.

Duration: Practice this Mudra for 15 minutes daily. For chronic kidney-related problems, practice this Mudra for 45 minutes every day. You can also split this up by practicing it for 15 minutes, thrice a day.

Benefits: This Mudra works at regulating any kidney disorders one might have. In addition to regulating kidney disorders, practicing this Mudra regularly can clear out blocked or running nose, pacify throat pain, and reduce swelling.

Note: Practice this Mudra in combination with Apana Mudra and Shank Mudra to release toxins and improve liver functionalities.

PRITHVI MUDRA

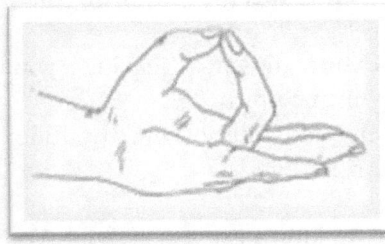

Instructions:
-Join the tips of your thumb and ring fingers.
-Stretch and straighten out the remaining three fingers such that they point upwards.

Duration: Practice this Mudra for 15 minutes, every day.

Benefits: As the name suggests the Prithvi Mudra works at balancing the earth element in the body. Practicing this Mudra regularly can increase vitality and strength. In this Mudra, we boost our immune system and with it, strengthen our bones, hair follicles, cartilages and skeleton structure.

Note: In addition to regulating the vitality and strength of the body, this Mudra helps cure jaundice, pacify fever and control hair loss.

SHANK MUDRA

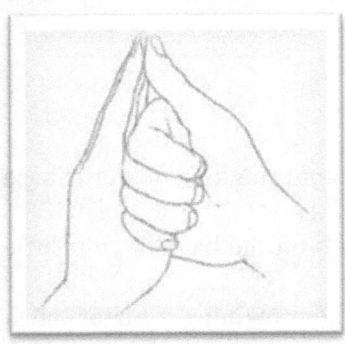

Instructions:
-Tuck your left thumb at the base of your right thumb. Now, fold the fingers of your right hand and cover your left thumb.
-Join the tip of your left index finger to the tip of your right thumb.
-Cradle the remaining three fingers of the left hand on the back of your right palm. (At this point, the formation should resemble a conch)

Duration: Practice this Mudra for 15 minutes, every day.

Benefits: Symbolic to its name, this Mudra resembles the shape of a conch and is hence called the "Shank Mudra". This Mudra regulates any imbalance in the thyroid gland. Practicing it regularly can help control obesity and pacify problems with voice larynx and throat.

Note: As this Mudra focuses on the well-being of the throat and voice larynx, it proves to be an effective voice therapy for aspiring singers!

Chapter 5 - Mudras for Specific Pains and Dis-Ease

BACK MUDRA

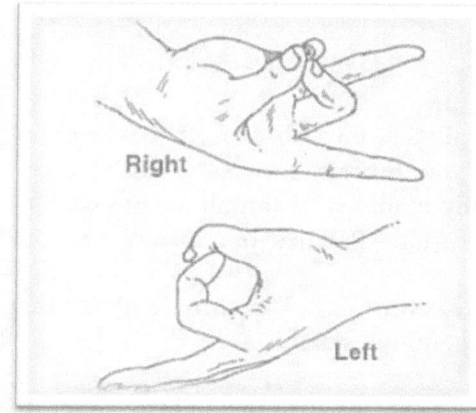

Instructions:
-Join the tips of your right thumb, middle and little fingers together while straightening open the remaining 2 fingers of your right hand.
-Next, join the tip of your left thumb to the tip of your left index finger.
-Stretch and straighten the remaining three fingers such that they point upwards.

Duration: Practice this Mudra for 15 minutes, every day. For chronic back aches, practice this Mudra for 45 minutes daily.

Benefits: We all know how excruciatingly painful a back ache can be. Often, we end up dousing ourselves with medicines and expensive treatments, only to have the pain resurfacing in quick time. _What if there was a way to relieve the pain and prevent it from resurfacing again?_ Well, the answer to this question lies in practicing the "back Mudra"!

Mudra for abdominal disorders and pains

MATANGI MUDRA

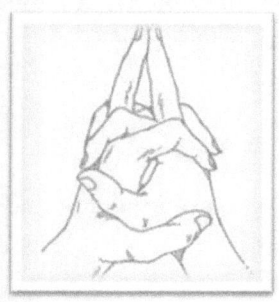

Instructions:
-Bring your palms together, clasping your fingers and drawing them in front of your stomach.
-Now, release your middle fingers such that they loosely touch each other's tips. (At this point, the remaining 8 fingers (excluding the 2 middle fingers) should be clasped together with your middle touching each other at the tips.)
Duration: Practice this Mudra for 15 minutes, every day. For chronic abdominal disorders or ailments, practice this Mudra for 45 minutes daily.

Benefits: This Mudra works at re-aligning breathing impulses in the solar plexus (stomach area) and redirects energy to heal and pacify any abnormalities in this area. Practicing this Mudra regularly can relieve chronic abdominal cramps and pacify any disorders that reside within it. In addition to the stomach area, this Mudra also works at regulating organs such as the kidney, pancreas, gallbladder, liver and spleen.

MUSHTI MUDRA

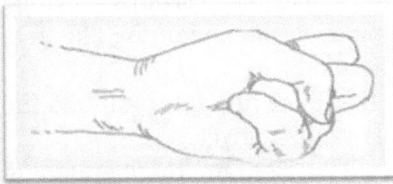

Instructions:
-Fold your fingers inwards such that they touch the base of your inner palm.
-Now, gently cradle your thumb on the back of your ring finger. (Practice this Mudra on both hands)

Duration: Practice this Mudra for 15 minutes, every day. For chronic abdominal disorders or ailments, practice this Mudra for 45 minutes daily.

Benefits: This Mudra works at regulating any abnormalities in the digestive tract. In addition to aiding better digestion, this Mudra helps relieve constipation and promote intestinal health.

SUCHI MUDRA

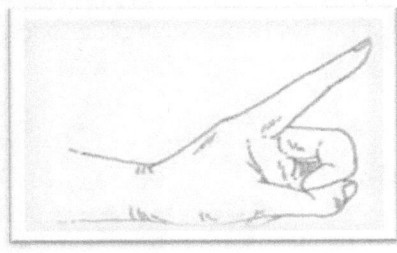

Instructions:
-Clench your fists together, drawing them in front of your chest.
-Now, inhale deeply and stretch out your right arm while pointing your index finger upwards. (At this point, the formation should resemble you pointing your index finger upwards. Note that the remaining 4 fingers of your right hand stay clenched in a fist.)
-Hold your breath for six counts.
-On the sixth count, gently release your fingers open.
-Repeat the steps on your left hand.

Duration: Practice this Mudra for 15 minutes, every day. For chronic abdominal disorders or ailments, practice this Mudra for 45 minutes daily.

Benefits: The Suchi Mudra works wonders at eliminating toxins and cleansing the abdominal region. This Mudra promotes intestinal cleaning, pacifies gastric activity, and eliminates prolonged constipation and abdominal cramps.

Mudras for circulatory disorders or heart-related problems

AAKASH MUDRA

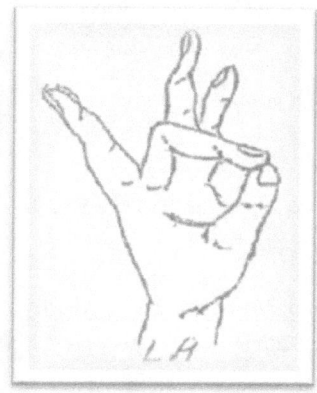

Instructions:
-Join the tips of your thumbs to the tips of your middle fingers.
-Stretch and straighten out your hands such that they point upwards.

Duration: Practice this Mudra for 15 minutes, every day. For chronic abdominal disorders or ailments, practice this Mudra for 45 minutes daily.

Benefits: Aakash symbolizes space; hence this Mudra works at regulating the space within the body. Increasing the space that resides between the four elements in the body gives each element the room it needs to thrive and act as needed. One of the main benefits of this Mudra is its ability to cure and pacify all heart-related problems. In addition to this, practicing this Mudra regularly aids detoxification, relives sinusitis and pacifies bone-relates disorders. On a mental and emotional level, this Mudra reduces inner conflict, depression, anger and aggression. While on the spiritual level, it aids self-realization and spiritual enlightenment!

GANESHA MUDRA

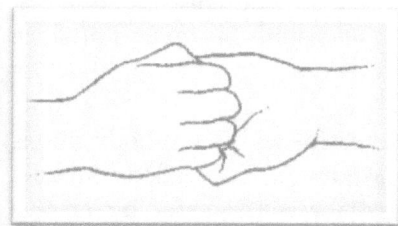

Instructions:
-Inhale and interlace the fingers of your hands such that they are clasped to their twin fingers on the other hand.
-Draw your interlaced fingers to the height of your heart such that they are stretched on opposite sides, horizontally.
-Hold your breath for 2 counts and stretch your hands in the opposite direction. Feel the tension build-up as you stretch them.
-Exhale, feel the tension ease out and relax.

Duration: Practice this Mudra for 15 minutes, every day. For chronic abdominal disorders or ailments, practice this Mudra for 45 minutes daily.

Benefits: Christened after Lord *Ganesha*, the God who is known to eliminate obstacles, this Mudra promotes and regulates the heart chakra. It helps open up the bronchial tubes, stimulating better blood circulation in the process. It also helps reduce feelings of fear, depression, anger and is an effective method to relieve any sort of heart related problems

Note: In addition this, we suggest you include Apana-Vayu Mudra, Linga Mudra, Prana Mudra, and Surya Mudra for a stronger and healthier heart!

SAMANA OR MUKULA MUDRA

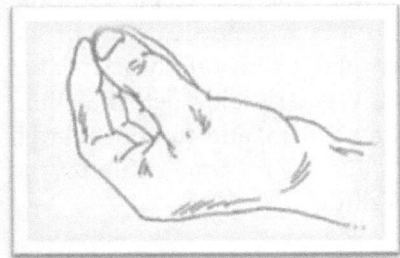

Instructions:
-Join the tip of your four fingers to the tip of your thumb.
-Next, place it on the point that's causing discomfort or pain. Conversely, you can also place it on your stomach for better digestion.
-Simultaneously, repeat this Mudra on the other hand.

Duration: Practice this Mudra for fifteen minutes daily. For chronic ailments, practice this Mudra for 45 minutes every day. You can also split this up and practice it for 15 minutes, thrice a day.

Benefits: "Samana" is one of the life-force energies that reside within our body, and is known to aid digestion. Resembling a bud, this Mudra is also called "Mukula Mudra". In this Mudra, you amalgamate the five energy forces (triggered by our five fingers) to come together in balance. Placing this Mudra on the point you have pain can instantly relieve the pain and rejuvenate any discomfort from it.

Mudras for nervous disorders

SHAKTI MUDRA

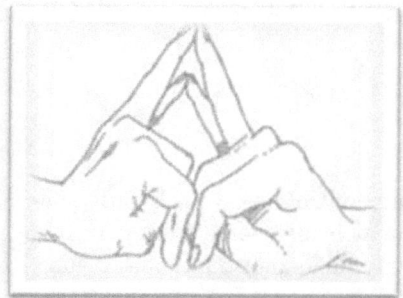

Instructions:
-Clasp your hands together, drawing them to the height of your heart.
-Inhale; curl the middle and index finger around the thumb loosely.
-Next, gently incline and join the tips of your right ring and little finger to the tips of your left ring and little finger. Hold your breath for as long as you can.
-Exhale and release the fingers open.

Duration: Practice this Mudra for 15 minutes, every day. For chronic sleeping disorders or nervousness, practice this Mudra for 45 minutes daily (preferably before you go to bed or are feeling most nervous.) You can also split this up by practicing it for 15 minutes, thrice a day.

Benefits: The Shakti Mudra soothes nerves and instills a calming effect on it. It helps regulate irregular sleep patterns while pacifying any restlessness in the mind. Practicing this Mudra regularly can see you experience longer periods of inner peace and contentment.

Note: In addition to the above Mudra, Jnana Mudra and Prithvi Mudra work wonders at calming down and pacifying any nervous disorders.

Mudra for longevity of life

DHARANA SHAKTI MUDRA

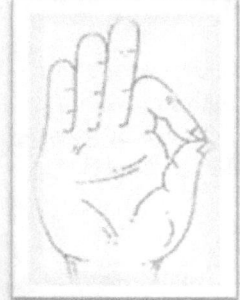

Instructions: This Mudra is practiced in three stages
In the first stage,
-Inhale and press the tip of your thumb to the tip of your index finger.
-Hold your breath for as long as you can. Note that this step of the Mudra prolongs breath control, allowing you to hold your breath for longer periods of time.
-Exhale and relax.

In the second stage,
-Inhale and press the middle of your thumb to the tip of your index finger.

-Hold your breath for as long as you can. Note that this step of the Mudra increases your control and hold on your breathing patterns.
-Exhale and relax.
In the final stage,
-Inhale and press the base of your thumb to the tip of your index finger. Hold your breath for as long as you can. Note that by this stage, you should be able to hold your breath for the longest time.
-Exhale and relax.

<u>Duration</u>: Practice this Mudra in five sets, every day.

<u>Benefits</u>: Dharana infers "retention". When you retain control over your breath, you gain the power to regulate the direction of your "Prana" or life -force energy. In the end, the longer your breath is the more control you have on its movement inside your body and the more energy it pumps into your organs. Practicing this Mudra regularly reduces increases the length of each breath and reduces the total number of breaths inhaled and exhaled in a day. This ultimately leads to higher energy levels and longevity of life.

Mudras for breathing disorders

BRONCHIAL MUDRA

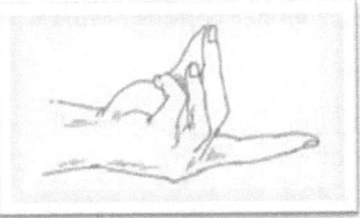

Instructions:
-Tuck your little finger at the base of your thumb.
-Place your ring finger on the soft spot of your thumb (mid thumb).
-Next, place your middle finger on the tip of your thumb.
-Stretch and straighten your index finger such that it points outwards.
-Hold this position for fifteen minutes while concentrating on regulating your breathing patterns.

<u>Duration</u>: Practice this Mudra for fifteen minutes or as long as you want.

<u>Benefits</u>: Synonymous to its name, this Mudra works wonders on the respiratory system and is also known as "Asthma Mudra". Practicing this Mudra regular can clear a blocked nose, stabilize irregular breathing patterns and relieve asthmatic attacks.

SHOONYA MUDRA
Instructions:

-Curl your middle finger to the base of your thumb.
-Next, gently cradle your thumb on the back of your middle finger.
-Stretch and straighten out the remaining three fingers such that they point outwards.
-Practice this Mudra on both hands for fifteen minutes.

Duration: Practice this Mudra for fifteen minutes. For chronic hearing disorders or ear infections, practice this Mudra for 45 minutes. You can also split this up and practice it for 15 minutes, thrice a day!

Benefits: This Mudra works at regulating the "ether or space element" in our body. Practicing this Mudra regularly can heal hearing disorders, relive irregular breathing patterns, cure ear infections and pacify vertigo symptoms.

Mudra to overcome bad habits

KALESVARA MUDRA

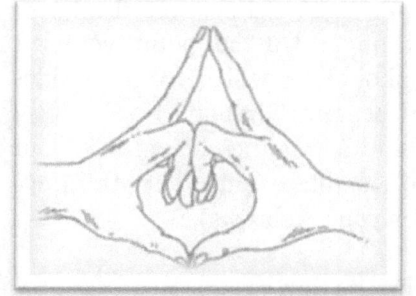

Instructions:
-Bring your hands close to each other, maintaining a small distance between them. Draw them to the height of your chest.
-Join the tips of your middle fingers.
-Curl your index fingers such that they join each other at their first joints.
-Similarly, curl your ring and little fingers such that they join each other at their first joints.
-Bring your thumbs forward and towards your chest such that they touch each other's tips.
-Meditate on your resolve to change and visualize it manifest in front of you.
-Observe your breathing patterns by inhaling and exhaling slowly.

Duration: Practice this Mudra for fifteen minutes or as long as you want!

Benefits: The Kalesvara Mudra is a powerful Mudra that helps transfigure the desire to change into reality. Practicing this Mudra regularly reinstates determination while instilling focus to eliminate bad habits. Practice this Mudra for fifteen minutes or longer periods and watch it transcend your resolutions into reality!

Note: As this Mudra also works at soothing the mind, it can be practiced as an effective tool to pacify nervous disorders.

Mudra for greater sexual health

KUNDALINI MUDRA

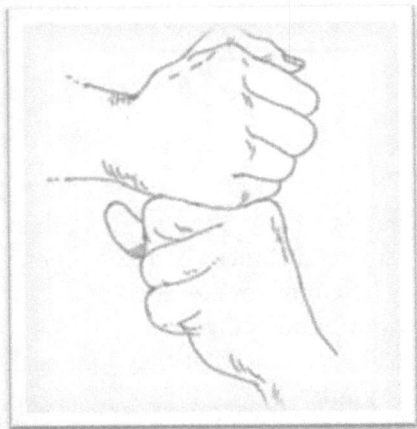

Instructions:
-Extend the index finger of your left hand while forming a fist with the remaining 4 fingers.
-Now, cover the left index finger with the index, middle, ring and little fingers of your right hand. Place your right thumb over the tip of your left index finger. (At this point, your left index fingers should be sealed from all sides with the fingers of your right hand.)
-Draw this Mudra to the height of your abdomen and meditate on your third-eye (region between your eyebrows).

Duration: Practice this Mudra for fifteen minutes, thrice a day!

Benefits: This Mudra symbolizes the "unison of the male and female force" and is associated with the reproductive energy. Practicing this Mudra regularly aids greater harmony between couples, leading to the birth of a new life.

Chapter 6 – Mudras for Mental Stability

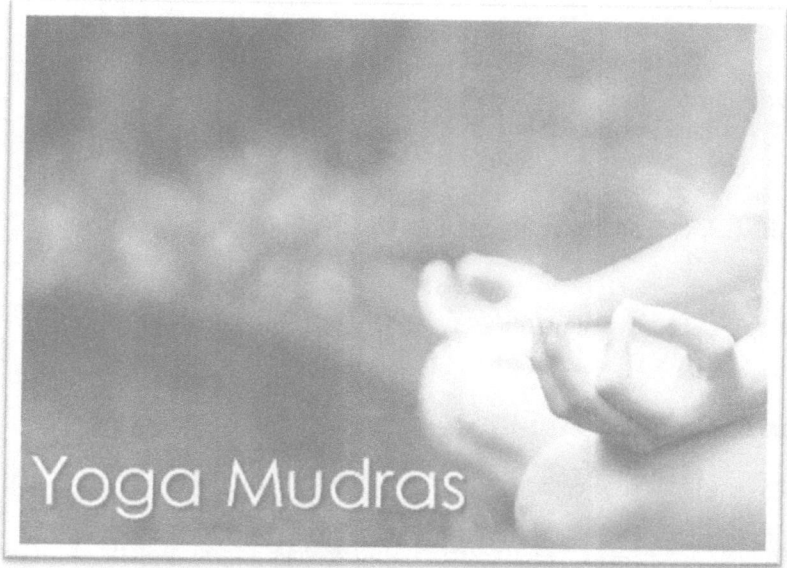

Source: http://3.bp.blogspot.com/-NWaIUo9KswA/UqB_C_-mqxI/AAAAAAAAEAI/FkOQAIZSik8/s1600/Mudras.png

When you are mentally or emotionally healthy, you are likely to have longer periods of "happy-time" and "inner-peace": a state where YOU drive the forces that control your emotions and behavior! However, being mentally balanced doesn't merely infer the absence of mental health problems, or that you are free of depression, anxiety and other psychological issues. Conversely, when you are mentally balanced, YOU exhibit characteristics that are POSITIVE and POWERFUL!

Practicing Mudras that aid mental and emotional stability can transcend you to a state where you're able to handle life's problems with ease, develop stronger relationships and recover quickly from any setbacks! In this section, I've carefully hand-picked Mudras that work at benefitting every aspect of your mental and emotional life. They guarantee a mood-boost even they build resilience and character to your overall personality. Practicing these Mudras diligently can give you the most rewarding experience, where YOU stay in control over how and what you want to feel!

Happy in Fifteen Minutes!

"Pain, loss, ailments, loneliness and death": these are a part of our life experiences. They help us evolve and make us the people we are today! Without anything to learn from, our evolution would remain stagnate, dissolving the very purpose of our existence!

Here, I've put forth some quick tips to help you address any emotional turbulence you might be going through:

-Think of every emotionally-draining experience as a learning curve in your life!
What is your pain today? What is it trying to teach you?

-Rewind the clock!
What are you doing to repeatedly invite this experience into your life?

-Think of a solution and address the problem head-on!
Ok, so how do you get yourself out of this vicious cycle?

-Follow and implement your positive thoughts!
Practice the below Mudras for 15 minutes and meditate on the resolve to fulfill your positive life-plan!

It's time to realize your inner POWER!

Mudras for mental stability

PALA MUDRA

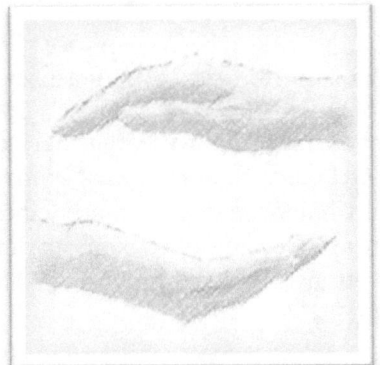

Instructions:
-This Mudra has to be practiced in a sitting position. First, cup your left hand with your palm facing upwards and place it just below your naval region.
-Next, inversely cup your right hand with your palm facing downwards and place it just below your chest region. (At this point, the formation should bracket the regions of your heart and stomach.)

Duration: Practice this Mudra for fifteen minutes every day. (Preferably at a time when you are feeling most stressed)

Benefits: "Pala Mudra" is known for its positive effects on the mind. It promotes clarity of thought, relieves stress and reduces anxiety. When practiced regularly, this Mudra reduces your thoughts per second (TPS), leaving you feeling mentally balanced and in-control!

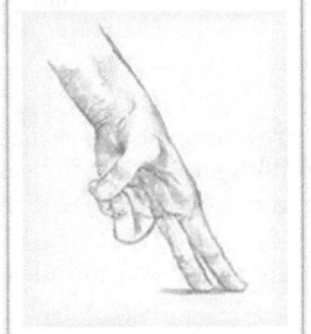

BHU MUDRA
Instructions:
-Staying seated, curl the little and ring fingers around the base of your thumb.

-Gently cradle your thumb on the back of your little and ring fingers.
-Next, extend and flex your middle and index fingers straight such that they form an inverted "V" shape.
-Finally, stretching your arms to the sides of your lap, touch the tips of your middle and index fingers (positioned in an inverted "V" shape) to the ground.

Duration: Practice this Mudra for fifteen minutes every day!

Benefits: "Bhu Mudra", also known as the "gesture of the earth" brings about a sense of stability in both, mind and body. This Mudra channelizes your life energies to remain in the "present" and "inside" your body. Practicing this Mudra regularly can reduce unnecessary inner chatter, mental conflict and uneasiness. What's more, practicing this Mudra for as less as 15 minutes every day can help you stay grounded and mentally balanced!

GARUDA MUDRA

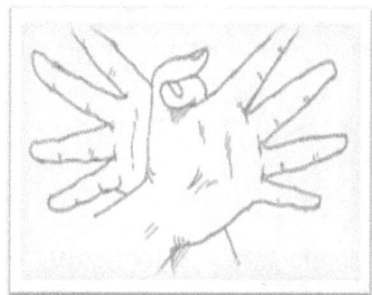

Instructions:
-Cradle the inside of your right palm on the back of your left palm.
-Intertwine and lock your thumbs such that the hand gesture symbolizes the two wings of a bird.
-Place your hands on your stomach for 5 minutes. Meditate on any uneasiness you might feel in this position and will it to free you.
-Next, place your hands close to your chest region for 10 minutes. Meditate on any uneasiness you might feel in this position and will it to free you.
-Relax and revel in the newly acquired freedom!

Duration: Practice this Mudra for 15 minutes every day. You can also practice it for longer periods or as long as you want!

Benefits: "Garuda" is a sacred mystical bird in Hindu mythology and hence, the "Garuda Mudra" works at regulating the space element in the body. In this Mudra, we create a sense of wide open space that helps free our mind from mental stress and worries. Practicing this Mudra regularly can help elevate moods, balance the mind, pacify the heart and fight exhaustion.

HAKINI MUDRA

Instructions:
-In this Mudra, join the tips of your left fingers with the tips of your right fingers,

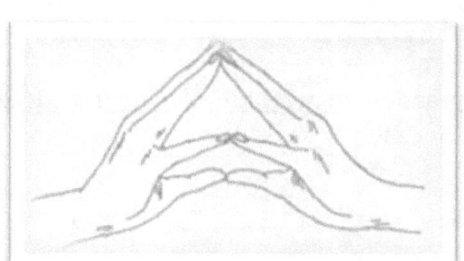

drawing your hands to the height of your chest.
-Fix your line of sight upwards.
-Inhale and place the tip of your tongue on top of your gums.
-Exhale and bring the tongue back to its original position.
-Repeat this Mudra for 15 counts or as long as you want.

Duration: Practice this Mudra for 15 minutes or longer periods.

Benefits: Inadvertently, this Mudra is quite common. You'll often notice people holding this positing when they are in deep contemplation or are trying to communicate a message across. In fact, it's even seen as a gesture that emulates confidence, intelligence and clarity of thought. Well, rightfully so; as this Mudra works at regulating aspects of your brain, making it sharper and clearer than ever before. Practicing this Mudra regularly can increase your memory power, instil clarity and mental stability.

RUDRA MUDRA

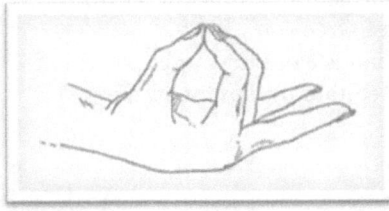

Instructions:
-Sit down in a comfortable position with your chest and chin held high.
-Inhale and exhale deeply.
-Take a few minutes to calm your mind and bring it to center. (At this point, you should be free of inner chatter and wavering thoughts.)
-Now, join the tips of your index and ring fingers to the tip of your thumb.
-Stretch and straighten your middle and little fingers such that they point outwards.
-Hold this position for fifteen minutes and release your fingers.
Duration: Practice this Mudra for fifteen minutes.

Benefits: The "Rudra Mudra" regulates the "earth element" in the body. In this Mudra, we regulate energies that flow through our Solar Plexus and mind. One of the primary benefits of this Mudra is its ability to stabilize the mind and bring in clarity. In addition to this, practicing this Mudra regularly helps relieve vertigo, dizziness, breathlessness, high blood pressure and poor eyesight.

Note: In addition to the above Mudras, practice Jnana Mudra, Samana Mudra, Kalesvara Mudra and Apana Mudra for superior mental health!

Chapter 7 – Mudras for Spiritual Possibilities

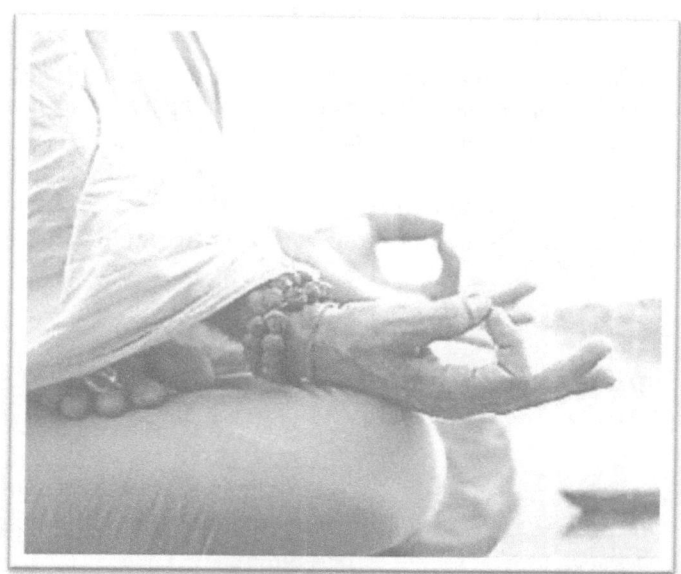

Source: https://yogamarrakech.files.wordpress.com/2011/06/Mudra2.jpg

Once there lived a fish, who along with other fish, swam and thrived in a pond. The pond was small and reflected a crowded, dark and gloomy ambience. While the other fish grumbled about the rather dark and unhappy ambience, our fish dreamt of ways to live in the light. He believed there was love and happiness, if only we were open and willing enough to invite it.

One day, after a quick lunch, the fish as usual tucked himself into a small corner and slipped into his dreams. He jumped out of the pond and followed the sun. First, he was nervous and anxious as hell, but his desire to see the light within and explore inner peace kept him going. He followed the light in his heart and travelled along the path it directed.

Little did he know that the journey would be as tough as it seemed. Suddenly, like a pack of cards crumbling down, he was left to deal with his inner most fears. He was forced to re-live every aspect of the past that troubled him. "This is more real than it had been before", he thought; as he willed himself to see the end of the journey!

Just when he stared at his darkest secret and saw it for the ultimate truth, he had refused to accept until then, he came across a great sea. The sea was a clear blue reflection of the sky above, it smelt fresh and wonderful. "This sea is big enough to house all the fish in the world", he thought!

His vision grew bigger and deeper, he now saw the trees that rustled at a distance, saw the sun shine brightly in front of him, he saw happiness and joy in everything he witnessed, every experience he lived! Our little fish had dived into the sea of enlightenment and was transformed! He had accessed his higher self! He opened his eyes and noticed that he had jumped into the great sea of "nothingness"! He had met with his higher self! Now, he held no ego and felt no remorse. Nothing worried him anymore: the lack of space, the thirst to know what's on the other side of the pond: nothing!

While he saw the other fish grumble about the lack of space, sunlight and hygiene in the pond, he swam through the great sea of inner peace and happiness! Our fish had found the sun within! He was spiritually transformed and enlightened!

Just as the fish, we too have a hidden spiritual self that needs to be awakened. The following Mudras work at re-aligning your energies in pursuit of higher spiritual awakening!

Mudras for spiritual ascension
SHANMUKHI MUDRA

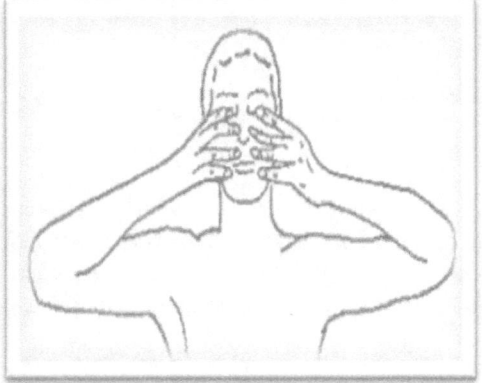

Instructions:
-Sit with your back held straight, drawing your elbows to the height of your shoulders.
-Plug in your thumbs inside your ears to block all external sounds.
-Close your eyes and use your index fingers to block your vision. (At this point, you should either see a combination of the rainbow colors.)
-Close your nostrils with your middle fingers to block your sense of smell.
-Caution: DO NOT block your nostrils completely and continuously. Make sure you leave enough room to breathe normally!
-Seal your lips with your ring and little fingers to block speech.
-Once you've isolated your six senses, Inhale and observe your breathing patterns. Listen to the vibrations it reverberates inside.
-Exhale and visualize the air travelling through the throat. Listen to the vibrations it reverberates inside.
-Feel the rainbow of colors swim through your body, give in to the calmness within and surrender to the divine energy that flows within you!
-Repeat this Mudra in between short intervals and experience it transcend you to a whole new spiritual dimension!

Suggested tips: The following fingers help shutting out the six sensory gates I spoke about earlier:
-The thumbs isolate sensations in the ears.

-The index fingers isolate sensations in the eyes.
-The middle fingers isolate sensations in the nose.
-The ring and little fingers isolate sensations inside the mouth.

Duration: Practice this Mudra for 20 minutes or longer periods.

Benefits: The "Shanmukhi Mudra" symbolizes "closing of the six gates or six senses". By practicing this Mudra, we consciously shut out our mind to the six senses namely, "our eyes, ears, nose and mouth", such that we steer clear of external distraction and stay focused on our inner state. In this Mudra, we focus on our breathing patterns to realize the light that resides within!

Note: In addition to the above Mudra, practice Jnana Mudra and Chin Mudra for spiritual ascension!

DHYANA MUDRA

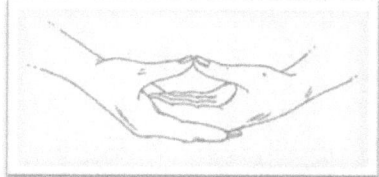

Instructions:
-Sit in a comfortable meditative pose. Observe your breathing patterns and meditate on your energy chakras.
-When in meditation, cradle your right palm over the left, with its inner sides facing upwards, and thumb touching each other.
-Stay thankful for all that you have and gradually surrendering to the divine energy that exists around us.
Duration: Practice this Mudra for 20 minutes or longer periods.

Benefits: The Dhyana Mudra is one of the first positions to adapt while meditating. Symbolizing the shape of an empty bowl, this Mudra implies our openness to learn and receive energy. Practicing this Mudra regularly will help us stay humble and receptive to the divine energy.

BHUMISPARSHA MUDRA

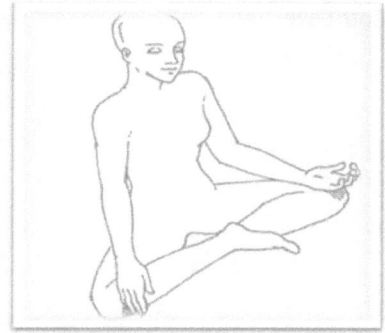

Instructions:
-Sit in a comfortable meditative pose. Observe your breathing patterns and meditate on your inner feelings.
-When in meditation, gradually slip the left hand down, with your fingers touching the ground.

-Now slip your right hand to the side with your fingers pointing upwards.
-Relax and experience the divine energy flow through every cell in your body!

Duration: Practice this Mudra for 20 minutes or longer periods.

Benefits: The "Bhumisparsha Mudra" is symbolic to the moment of the Buddha's awakening! Practicing this Mudra regularly will lead us to the path of "true happiness", where we realize the purpose of our being!

NAGA MUDRA

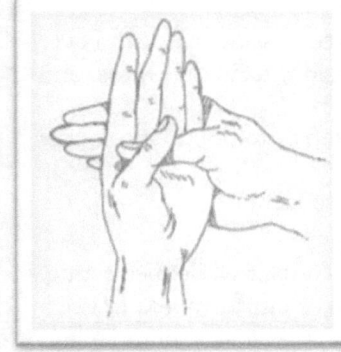

Instructions:
-Cradle your right palm on the back of your left.
-Bring your right thumb forward and place it at the base of your left index finger.
-Next, cradle your left thumb on the back of your right thumb such that they intersect each other.

Duration: Practice this Mudra for 20 minutes or longer periods.

Benefits: The journey to spiritual growth is no different from the one we encounter every day. Just as we encounter obstacles in our physical life, we will have to encounter and overcome worldly challenges in our spiritual path. Christened after the Hindu snake god "Naga", this Mudra symbolizes supernatural strength, wisdom and power. In this Mudra, we gain access to our higher self and can seek answers from within. Hence, this Mudra is also called "the Mudra of deeper knowledge". Practicing this Mudra regularly will give us the insight we need to solve every day problems and pursue spiritual growth.

Mudras for manifestation

KUBERA MUDRA

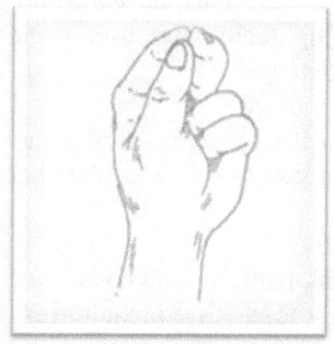

Instructions:
-Curl the ring and little fingers of your hand to the base of your palm.
-Next, join the tip of your index and middle fingers to the tip of your thumb.
-Holding this position in both hands for 20 minutes or more can help bring your energy circuits together and activate your Kundalini.
Duration: Practice this Mudra for 20 minutes or longer periods!

Benefits: The Kubera Mudra is a Mudra that helps manifest your dreams into reality. Practicing this Mudra regularly can see you invite abundance health, prosperity and happiness into your life!

Note: Within the first five minutes into this Mudra, you'll notice a reverberating energy field around the tips of your fingers. If this energy is too strong to hold, release your hands and start over again after a short break.

SURABHI MUDRA

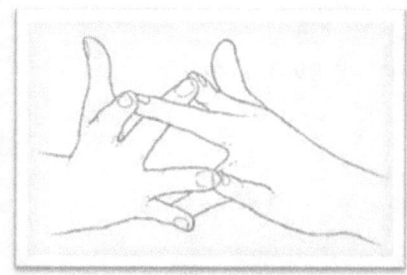

Instructions:
-Clasp your hands together in Anjali or Namaste Mudra with your thumb inching apart.
-Next, join the tip of your left index finger to the tip of your right middle finger.
-Similarly, join the tip of your right index finger to the tip of your left middle finger.
-Now, join the tip of your right ring finger to the tip of your left little finger.
-Similarly, join the tip of your left ring finger to the tip of your right little finger.

Duration: Practice this Mudra for twenty minutes or longer periods!

Benefits: The "Surabhi Mudra", similar to the "Kubera Mudra" is a Mudra that helps manifest your dreams into reality. In addition to fulfilling desires and dreams, practicing this Mudra regularly promotes better functionality of the pituitary, adrenaline and thyroid glands.

Conclusion and Next Steps

Practicing Mudras as a way of life

Mudras are the perfect tools for superior physical health and spiritual elevation. These subtle movements, in combination with breathing techniques and yogic exercises can help us discover the higher purpose of our existence!

In this book, I've focused on the physical, mental and spiritual benefits of Mudras. However, in addition to practicing Mudras, I gently urge you to follow a diet that promotes, maintains and restores a "*Sattvic*" way of life.

The word "*Sattvic*" infers all that is pure, natural, essential, truthful, and conscious! Consuming a moderate diet that is balanced with seasonal foods that include fresh fruits, dairy products, nuts, seeds, oils, ripe vegetables, pulses, whole grains, and non-meat-based-proteins can help you nurture a body that is ready for longevity, physical health and spiritual awakening!

On that note, I urge you to do whatever it takes to practice the Mudras every day. This is the all-important step that will enable you to produce the results you're committed to: a promise you have to make to yourself!

Let your journey begin!

Thank you for downloading this book. I've had a profound healing experience writing it and believe this experience will transfer to you, my reader.

If you enjoyed this book, I'd greatly appreciate your review on Amazon.

~ Diane Clarke

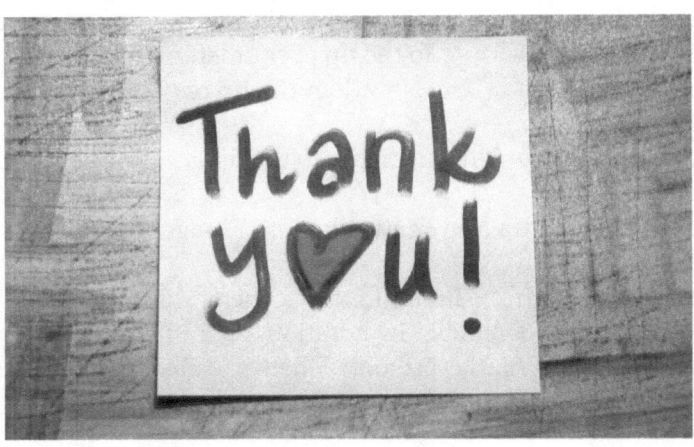